HEAL YOUR CHAKRAS

ENERGY AWARENESS SERIES

ALEXA ISPAS

WORD BOTHY

CONTENTS

INTRODUCTION

Welcome to this amazing journey of self-discovery.

It is my honor to guide you as you learn how to heal your chakras.

Throughout this book, I will take a practical approach.

The book will answer questions such as, to what extent is the energy in your chakras vibrant and flowing well?

In which chakra(s) is your energy stuck, and in what way?

Is there too much, or too little energy in a particular chakra?

Your chakras are like a mini orchestra inside your body, composed of seven different instruments.

These seven instruments cover the whole of your life.

They range from the most material aspects of life, covered by your root chakra, to the most spiritual, which are related to your crown chakra.

When your chakras are balanced and working well, it's as if your entire being is making the most harmonious and enticing music you could ever imagine.

You have probably had moments in your life when you experienced perfect harmony.

Everything flowed easily, and you were able to deal with anything that came your way in a balanced and graceful way.

On the other hand, most of the time, this is probably not the case.

If you are like most people, one or more of your chakras is out of balance on a regular basis.

When this is the case, there is either too little energy flowing through the chakra (it is underactive) or there is too much energy in that center (it is overactive).

At such times, your mini orchestra is still making music, but the instruments aren't working well together.

If this is your current situation, you are prob-ably not living out your full potential.

You may also have encountered times in your life when nothing was working.

At such times, it's like the instruments in your orchestra were playing different tunes.

In such cases, your whole life becomes an emergency.

The only way to sort things out is to slam the breaks.

Otherwise, every added step takes you closer to disaster.

Whatever situation you are currently in, I hope this book will help.

If you are currently enjoying a harmonious period of your life, reading this book will help you maintain this harmony long-term.

Through learning how to consciously work with your chakras, you will identify imbalances as they arise, instead of letting them become bigger and more destructive over time.

Or you may be in the second category and feel that things could be better.

You may feel stuck in a particular area of your life and not know how to get unstuck.

This book will enable you to identify exactly

what you need to address to bring every element of your life into a harmonious, enjoyable whole.

And finally, if you have recently had to slam the breaks, this book will provide you with the clarity to start re-building on a new, solid foundation.

In each chapter, we will focus on a particular chakra.

You will learn about the specific energy that is connected with that chakra.

You will also become able to recognize how that energy shows up when it is healthy and vibrant.

This will give you a 'baseline' as your point of reference.

You will then discover the 'essential problem' associated with that chakra when it is out of balance.

Each chakra has a specific way in which it gets distorted.

This essential problem shows up in one of two ways, depending on whether the chakra is underactive or overactive.

I have provided a list of symptoms for each as well as a more in-depth explanation, so you can assess whether that chakra is at either of these two extremes for you.

You may also find that one of your chakras is sometimes underactive and other times overactive, depending on the situation.

For example, the heart chakra often becomes underactive after a heartbreak, then swings to overactive once the loneliness becomes too difficult to bear.

This swing from one extreme to the other happens with most people.

Do not be alarmed if for some chakras, you identify both underactive as well as overactive aspects within yourself.

The key is to become conscious of the imbalance and of the extreme you are gravitating towards.

Once you are aware of these extremes and learn to recognize them, you will find it easier to bring yourself back to balance.

To do so, I have provided two exercises for each of the underactive/overactive extremes.

You can use these exercises to bring your chakras back to balance.

You can do the relevant exercises as you read the book, or you might like to do them once you have an overview of everything that is available to you.

I strongly suggest you do the exercises, as mental awareness can only go so far.

The exercises will ground your knowledge and make it 'present' for you in a way that simply being aware of your chakras theoretically cannot.

I have kept this book short, so you can read it over the course of a day and gain the practical tools to start healing your chakras straight away.

And now, without further ado, let us begin our journey.

ROOT CHAKRA

ABOUT YOUR ROOT CHAKRA

Your root chakra is located at the base of your spine.

Its energy also connects to your legs and your feet.

In the metaphorical sense (chakras are full of metaphorical language!), your feet are your 'roots', the foundation for the rest of your body.

The energy of your root chakra is about survival in the physical sense.

In addition, as the chakras deal with the subtle realm of existence, this chakra also relates to any beliefs you have about your right to occupy a space in this world.

Your root chakra is the foundation for your whole life.

If you have a strong foundation, you are likely to feel safe and secure, responding to whatever life throws at you with ease and grace.

A tree with deep, strong roots can withstand even the most severe storm.

In the same way, a person with a strong root chakra experiences an inner feeling of calm and safety no matter what is going on around them.

Your root chakra allows you to feel 'at home' in your body.

It enables you to relax in situations where there isn't any immediate threat.

This sense of being in tune with your body means you are likely to enjoy good health and vitality.

You are also likely to feel motivated and empowered to take care of your physical needs.

Your ability to find your way 'home', back to your roots, gives you a strong sense of trust in the world.

Your root chakra also gives you the ability to stand up for yourself in situations of conflict.

A person with a strong root chakra is not a pushover.

ROOT CHAKRA PROBLEMS

Problems with the root chakra generally stem from not feeling safe in the material world.

The issues relating to the root chakra are so basic that when things do not work at this level, it affects everything else.

The material world is in constant flux.

This can be difficult for your root chakra, as this chakra thrives on consistency and predictability.

How you deal with this state of flux has profound implications for the way you navigate life.

At the core of any root chakra imbalance is chronic fear.

Of course, fear is a useful emotion.

It motivates you to avoid unnecessary risks and therefore keeps you out of harm's way.

When only experienced occasionally and in situations that are dangerous, fear does not cause an imbalance.

The sense of safety provided by the root chakra returns as soon as the danger is over.

However, when your root chakra is out of

balance, what you are dealing with is not fear that arises out of a dangerous situation.

Instead, you are dealing with chronic fear.

This type of fear arises even though there is an absence of actual physical danger.

Chronic fear blocks the functioning of your root chakra.

It therefore prevents you from experiencing the enormous benefits the energy of a strong, healthy root chakra would bring into your life.

Fear can show up in different ways, depending on whether your root chakra is primarily underactive or overactive.

UNDERACTIVE ROOT CHAKRA

- Disconnecting from the body
- Anxious and restless
- Poor focus and discipline
- Financial difficulties
- Poor boundaries

When your root chakra is underactive, you are likely to feel that your life is built on a shaky foundation.

This sense of un-groundedness leads to a variety of coping mechanisms.

You may, for example, keep spinning your wheels yet not accomplish anything.

Your daily life may feel like a constant battle for survival.

Under such circumstances, even the most basic aspects of life feel difficult: taking care of your health, making money, even keeping a roof over your head.

Having an underactive root chakra makes you restless and unfocused.

This can have a negative impact on the way you deal with the material world.

You are likely to worry about your financial security, the possibility of being fired from your job, or your business failing.

It may feel that no matter how hard you try, you will never have enough money, time, or space to do the things that matter to you or that bring you pleasure.

You may also disconnect from your body without realizing.

This is because in the absence of your root chakra's calming energy, your body is likely to feel uncomfortable.

It is therefore tempting to disconnect from your body to avoid experiencing this discomfort.

The most common sign you are disconnecting from your body is that you do not take proper care of your body's needs.

For example, you may find yourself going long stretches of time without eating or moving your body.

This disconnection from your body may even show up while doing physical activities such as going to the gym.

Your way of disconnecting at such times may be to distract yourself from the signals your body is sending you.

For example, you might exercise with your headphones on, away in a world of your own, not paying attention to your body.

As your body is depleted of the strong, physical energy it needs to allow you to truly 'show up' in the world, it is often restless and jittery.

An ungrounded body, in turn, gives signals to others that you do not have the strength to stand your ground or maintain consistency.

As such, you may find yourself getting picked as a target by pushy, unscrupulous people.

This is likely to have a detrimental effect on your finances as well as your sense of self.

The longer this disconnection from your body goes on, the easier it gets for others to push you around.

You may frequently have to adapt to other people's agenda, while your own wishes are dismissed.

UNDERACTIVE ROOT CHAKRA HEALING

If your root chakra is underactive, the main priority is to reconnect with your body.

Doing so is a matter of learning how to stay connected to your body at all times, instead of trying to escape it at the slightest sign of discomfort.

The more you learn not to disconnect from your body when experiencing discomfort, the safer you will feel within yourself.

This sense of safety will be felt by those around you.

Over time, you will get better at asserting yourself and taking up your rightful place.

UNDERACTIVE ROOT CHAKRA EXERCISES

Massage your feet

One of the easiest ways to heal an underactive root chakra is to pay special attention to your feet.

Your feet are like the roots of a tree.

The more stable the roots, the healthier the tree.

The way to create this sense of stability is to make sure your feet are connected to the ground and there is lots of energy flowing through them.

Give yourself a foot massage once a day, or as often as possible.

Make the foot massage as vigorous as you can without hurting yourself, to get the energy moving.

This energy will then flow through the rest of your body, spreading the calming vibration of your root chakra throughout.

If you don't enjoy foot rubs, even simply becoming aware of your feet will start healing your root chakra.

Pay attention to the way you position your feet throughout your day.

For example, are your feet firmly planted on the ground, or are they moving about while you are talking to someone?

If you regularly wear high heels, try not wearing them for a while, or at least give yourself lots of heel-free time.

Notice the effect this has on your inner sense of safety.

Engage your body in dialogue

The basic idea behind this exercise is that your body is made up of different parts, like an orchestra is made up of different instruments.

Each part of your body therefore has a voice.

It has things to say that are worth hearing.

Some parts of your body may have positive messages for you, while others may tell you about their difficulties.

This exercise will allow you to communicate with different parts of your body.

You will begin to hear and become acquainted with the multiplicity of voices that are alive inside you.

In doing so, you will help any painful areas in your body transmute stuck energy.

You will also get in touch with the needs of your body on a day-to-day basis.

It is best to do this exercise at a time when you can fully relax.

You may also want to keep a journal and a pen next to you.

This is an optional part of the exercise, but I have found it helpful in my own practice.

Documenting your sessions in a journal allows you to analyze how the messages coming from different parts of your body are evolving over time.

To begin the exercise, close your eyes and direct your attention towards your body.

Now bring your attention to your feet.

Start imagining you *are* your feet.

If your feet were able to talk, what would they say? What is their experience of life?

For example, if I was doing the exercise just now, speaking as my feet, I would say, 'I want to wiggle'.

As I say this, I realize that my feet are quite stiff, and that I would like to wiggle them.

As I do so, I experience the joy in my feet as they start to wiggle.

It's like they are two mischievous school-children who have been sitting at their desk for too long and have just been allowed to run into the schoolyard and play.

If you are using a journal, you can record what your feet said when they were asked to speak, and how it felt when you acknowledged their wish.

You don't need to write much.

For example, you could write 'feet' and next to it 'we'd like to wiggle' and 'joyful'.

Or you could write a whole stream of consciousness on what your feet are experiencing.

Tailor this exercise to your needs. There is no right or wrong way of doing it.

Move your attention to your ankles.

Speaking as your ankles, what would you like to say?

You might then want to move on to your knees, your hips, your belly, and so on.

Consider if you would like to include your internal organs such as your liver and your kidneys.

You might want to do this exercise from the bottom up or start at the top of your body.

Once again, there is no right or wrong way.

There is only what feels right for you, and what you'd like to experiment with.

Aim to do this exercise regularly, for example once a day or once a week.

Keep journaling about it.

Over time you will start to get a detailed overview of what is going on in your body.

You may see patterns emerging, such as the left side of your body being more vocal than the right side, or the bottom of your body being less happy than the upper half.

You may also find that some body parts will try to get more of your attention.

Enjoy this exercise and keep experimenting with different ways of doing it.

OVERACTIVE ROOT CHAKRA

- Fear of change
- Addiction to security
- Rigid boundaries
- Obesity/overeating
- Hoarding/material fixation
- Sluggish and tired

When your root chakra is overactive, the way you deal with chronic fear is to resist change.

This is often accompanied by an overemphasis on the material aspects of life through behaviors such as overeating and hoarding.

Physically you may feel sluggish and tired due

to overeating.

Your body may be heavy set, and you might have trouble losing weight.

Your environment is also likely to reflect your resistance to change.

You might have difficulty letting go of clutter, and the energy in your living environment may feel heavy and stuck.

Your lower chakras may be so overactive that you have difficulty developing the gifts of your upper chakras, such as vision and trust in the Universe.

This is likely to become part of a vicious cycle.

The less you can envision the future, the more you resist change.

OVERACTIVE ROOT CHAKRA HEALING

If your root chakra is overactive, there is too much energy in this center.

To heal this imbalance, you need to start engaging with fresh ideas.

This will stimulate your upper chakras and lighten the energy in your root chakra.

You also need to engage with the uncertainty of change and release your attachment to security.

The more you step out of your comfort zone and experience success in doing so, the easier it will be to engage with novel situations.

OVERACTIVE ROOT CHAKRA EXERCISES

Engage with new ideas

Do you have anybody in your environment, perhaps your place of work, who brings in new ideas?

Try engaging them in discussion and asking them questions about their ideas.

Do not challenge them, simply listen to what they have to say and allow yourself time to consider their ideas.

To heal an overactive root chakra, you need to prioritize the subtle dimension of existence.

This includes opening up to new ideas and possibilities while lessening your focus on material things.

As your upper chakras become more active and bring in more fresh ideas to you, the material aspects of your life are likely to change.

For example, the new ideas may show you how to work less yet earn more, and generally put in less effort yet create a bigger impact.

If you have an overactive root chakra, reading this book is already a step in the right direction.

Keep opening yourself up to new ideas, and your root chakra will gradually rebalance itself.

Step out of your comfort zone

Ask yourself, how can you step out of your comfort zone?

If your life is repetitive and stagnant, allow serendipity and randomness to come in.

Break out of the rigid structure you have built up and see what you can do to introduce flow into your life.

Allow yourself to have new experiences and delight in all they have to offer.

Stepping out of your comfort zone forces you to let go of what you know and venture into the unknown.

This allows the dense, compacted energy in your root chakra to lighten.

At the same time, stepping out of your comfort zone strengthens your upper chakras.

These chakras thrive on problem-solving and learning how to deal with novel situations.

SACRAL CHAKRA

ABOUT YOUR SACRAL CHAKRA

Your sacral chakra is located around the area of your pelvis and genital organs.

Its energy also connects with the joints in your body.

The energy associated with this chakra is related to pleasure.

While discussing the root chakra, we have delved into the physical needs of your body.

With the sacral chakra we are going one step further, into what makes you *feel* good.

This is no longer about simply providing your body with the basics of life.

The energy of your sacral chakra takes you beyond surviving and into thriving.

A person with a healthy sacral chakra is fun to be around.

They know how to enjoy life and how to bring the 'fun factor' to those around them.

People with a healthy sacral chakra are enthusiastic and well-balanced emotionally.

They can soothe themselves when things don't go their way.

They express their uncomfortable emotions and then go back to having fun.

There is flexibility in their way of being, yet they are not pushovers.

Their physical movements are graceful, balanced, and full of unselfconscious sensuality.

SACRAL CHAKRA PROBLEMS

Problems with the sacral chakra generally stem from difficulty experiencing pleasure.

This difficulty is bound up with the underlying belief that pleasure has to be 'earned', or that it is in some way wrong to experience this feeling.

Due to this underlying belief, doing something

that elicits pleasure becomes bound up with guilt, which spoils the pleasurable feeling.

When the sacral chakra is out of balance long-term, this is due to a chronic feeling of guilt.

As with fear in the root chakra, guilt can be a useful emotion when experienced appropriately.

In such cases, feeling guilty after taking a particular action gives you the signal that in hindsight, you wish you had taken a different course.

As such, if the same situation were to repeat itself, you would act differently.

Chronic guilt, by contrast, means you experience this emotion whether you have done something wrong or not.

You may be experiencing guilt at the slightest things, such as having a critical thought about someone or eating a slice of cake.

When you are plagued by chronic guilt, life becomes a minefield of triggers that reinforce the guilt you are feeling.

As a result of having this uncomfortable emotional undercurrent, you are likely to resort to unhealthy coping mechanisms.

These coping mechanisms differ based on whether you have an underactive or an overactive sacral chakra.

UNDERACTIVE SACRAL CHAKRA

- Rigid body and attitude
- Poor social skills
- Low sex drive
- Denial of pleasure
- Lack of desire, passion, and excitement

If you have an underactive sacral chakra, you attempt to control your guilt by eliminating pleasure from your life.

This results in a lack of flexibility.

This can be seen, among other things, in the way you handle yourself physically.

Your body is likely to appear rigid.

This is because you don't have the flexibility and playfulness (in both body and attitude) that a healthy sacral chakra brings.

You may also be disinterested in sex or not have the energy for it.

At the emotional level, an underactive sacral chakra may show up as poor social skills.

This is due to the lack of playfulness that comes with rigidity.

Having social skills requires spontaneity and the ability to quickly respond to other people's opening gambits.

With an underactive sacral, you do not have the spontaneity for this kind of back-and-forth.

In general, people with an underactive sacral chakra tend to lack desire, passion, and excitement.

They aren't fun to be around and tend not to enjoy being around other people outside of a structured environment.

UNDERACTIVE SACRAL CHAKRA HEALING

If your sacral chakra is underactive, this means you have too little energy in this center.

To heal this imbalance, you need to bring in more energy into this area.

One way to do this is to make use of your sacral chakra's connection to movement.

This chakra is the most easily activated by movement in your body, particularly movement in the area of your hips and pelvis.

Get into the habit of regularly moving your body in ways you enjoy and that stimulate your hips and pelvis.

At a deeper level, to heal an underactive sacral chakra, you need to start becoming comfortable with pleasure.

This may be easier said than done and requires a change of mindset.

If your sacral chakra is underactive, it is likely that the concept of allowing yourself time for pleasure is alien to you.

However, the fact you are reading this book shows you are ready for this kind of deep mindset change.

I would therefore recommend you start at the beginning, with identifying the kinds of things that bring you pleasure.

This will encourage you to look for opportunities to allow pleasure into your life.

UNDERACTIVE SACRAL CHAKRA EXERCISES

Move your body

The easiest and quickest way to heal an underactive sacral chakra is to regularly wiggle your hips.

You can wiggle them any way feels comfortable to you.

If you need guidance on how to do it, watch a belly dancing clip online and you'll get the idea.

Alternatively, how about buying yourself a hula hoop and using it regularly?

Wiggling your hips is a wonderful way of getting energy moving through your sacral area.

This area is the most vulnerable part of your body.

It is common to tense up this area when anything uncomfortable arises in your environment or in your thoughts.

The more you can bring conscious attention to this area and keep it physically moving, the more energy will start flowing through it.

Try shaking your hips at least once a day, even just for one minute at a time, and see how much zest for life you'll start to find within yourself.

Identify what brings you pleasure

What brings you pleasure is highly individual.

You need to discover the things that bring *you* pleasure, away from any conditioning you may have received while growing up.

There are different kinds of pleasure: physical, emotional, intellectual, and spiritual.

You may be attracted to some more than others.

Physical pleasure is the kind of pleasure you feel in relation to your body.

It includes sexual pleasure, but it also arises when you do anything that involves your body and that you enjoy.

For example, many people experience this type of pleasure when they exercise.

Emotional pleasure often comes from connecting with someone, such as having a heart-to-heart with your best friend.

Intellectual pleasure often comes from learning new things or having intellectually stimulating discussions with others.

Spiritual pleasure arises when you take care of the needs of your soul.

Make a list of what brings you pleasure, and include some of these activities into your day.

OVERACTIVE SACRAL CHAKRA

- Binging
- Procrastination
- Addiction problems
- Obsessive attachment

If your sacral chakra is overactive, you attempt to override your chronic guilt by distracting yourself.

An overactive sacral chakra is associated with binging, procrastinating, or other behaviors where the pleasure-seeking gets out of control and turns into addiction.

The underlying problem is still the same as with an underactive sacral chakra: an inability to experience true pleasure, and therefore also an inability to fulfill your emotional needs.

However, in the case of an overactive sacral chakra, the inability to experience pleasure translates into an obsession with experiencing pleasure at all cost.

This extreme focus on pleasure often leads to addictive behaviors, as well as heightened emotionality and mood swings.

A healthy way of experiencing pleasure is to fulfill your need for something, then move on.

Pleasure allows you to enjoy things and let them go, honoring the constant flow of life.

By contrast, in the case of an overactive sacral chakra, addiction takes the place of pleasure.

The result is that you get stuck in a loop, with the emotional background to this loop being guilt.

The addiction loop looks something like this: I want something, because it would fulfill a genuine emotional need in me.

But due to the undercurrent of chronic guilt, having it is entangled with discomfort.

Once I have some, I want more, in the hope that I will feel pure pleasure without the discomfort.

But because of the chronic guilt, I cannot enjoy it.

This means I want it even more, motivated by the need to finally experience that feeling of pure pleasure.

As every time the pleasure is accompanied by guilt, I can never get that sense of completion I seek.

Can you see how insidious this loop is?

When you are stuck in this loop, you can never get enough.

As the guilt keeps piling up, you lose the ability to remain in charge of your feelings and actions.

OVERACTIVE SACRAL CHAKRA HEALING

To heal an overactive sacral chakra, you need to restore your relationship with pleasure.

This is likely to take a lot of time and practice.

The high emotional charge that accompanies an overactive sacral chakra makes it difficult to be disciplined.

However, every tiny step in the right direction is a step forward.

The first priority is to break the pattern of addictive behavior in your everyday life.

To do so, you need to identify your unmet emotional needs.

It is these needs that, due to being unmet, set the whole negative cycle in motion.

Therefore, it is worth consciously engaging with your unmet needs and finding healthy ways to meet them.

The other aspect of this healing process is training your body to recognize the difference between pleasure and addiction.

The more you become able to make that distinction, the earlier you will be able to sense when you are slipping into addictive behavior.

When you can see it coming, you are in a better position to break the cycle and shift your focus onto pleasurable alternatives.

OVERACTIVE SACRAL CHAKRA EXERCISES

Identify your unmet needs

Ask yourself, what unfulfilled emotional needs do you have?

How do your addictive behaviors help you cope with these unfulfilled needs?

Are there healthier ways to get these needs met?

Identify the underlying emotional needs fueling the addictive behavior, whether that is literally addiction or milder forms such as procrastination and binging.

This is likely to be difficult emotionally.

After all, the reason you are stuck in the addiction loop is to distract yourself from these unfulfilled needs.

However, as you are reading this book, you may be at a stage in your life where you feel motivated to address these needs.

If so, it may also be a good idea to find a therapist or someone who can help you through this journey.

You do not have to do everything on your own, especially this difficult stage of the process.

There is excellent help available if you look for it. Give yourself the opportunity to find it.

Once you have identified your underlying unfulfilled needs, you need to allow yourself time to heal and grieve for what is lost.

After that, it is time to satisfy these needs in healthier ways.

Finding alternative, healthy ways to satisfy deep unfulfilled emotional needs is likely to take a lot of creativity on your part.

This process takes practice and willpower.

You also need a healthy dose of self-compassion for those times when you choose to give in to your addictive tendencies.

After all, the reason you resorted to the addictive behavior in the first place is probably because the original need is difficult to satisfy.

However, with some careful self-analysis and perhaps professional help, you can find alternative ways to fulfill your emotional needs.

Reconnect with pleasure

Another piece of the puzzle for getting out of addictive patterns is to reconnect with the way it feels to experience pleasure.

To do so, find something that is pleasurable to you, but that is not subject to your addictive pattern.

This most likely involves something you do not feel the same intensity as what is fueling the addiction.

Instead, it is likely to have a subtler effect on you, one that allows you to feel pleasure in a quiet, contented way.

As you experience this pleasurable activity, start bringing your attention to your body.

What does it feel like to experience pleasure, as opposed to addiction?

Can you sense the difference?

It is important to give yourself lots of opportunities to experience the difference between pleasure and addiction, and to do this over an extended period.

The more you can sense the difference in your body between pleasure and addiction, the more you will start resonating with the feeling of pleasure.

You will also start recognizing the discomfort that is associated with addictive behavior.

This is an important step forward.

The more uncomfortable the addictive behavior becomes, the easier it gets to choose pleasurable over addictive activities.

SOLAR PLEXUS CHAKRA

ABOUT YOUR SOLAR PLEXUS CHAKRA

Your solar plexus chakra is located in your solar plexus area.

Its energy connects with your digestive organs.

The energy of your solar plexus chakra gives you access to your willpower and your sense of individual identity.

This is the chakra of taking action and asserting yourself in the world.

When you have a healthy solar plexus chakra, you feel confident within yourself.

The energy of this chakra gives you a sense that you are at the helm of your own destiny.

You know you always have a choice in the way you deal with whatever comes your way.

You are self-disciplined and have a strong work ethic, with excellent motivation and the willpower to see projects through to completion.

People with a healthy solar plexus chakra are also good at setting boundaries.

If conflict arises, they can stand their ground.

In the public sphere, they enjoy being visible and making a positive impact.

At the same time, they do not rely on other people's praise for their sense of self.

SOLAR PLEXUS CHAKRA PROBLEMS

Problems with the solar plexus chakra generally stem from a distorted sense of self.

The solar plexus chakra is about your solar identity.

This energy offers a coherent view of yourself.

Nobody questions the sun. It elicits respect and awe.

However, when there is an imbalance in your solar plexus chakra, your sense of self doesn't feel like the sun.

Instead, you feel insecure about yourself at a fundamental level.

This is often connected with chronic shame.

Guilt and shame are different emotions.

Guilt makes you feel bad about something you have done.

Shame makes you feel bad about yourself.

Guilt is about having made a mistake. Shame makes you think you *are* a mistake.

Feeling shame therefore leads to a much deeper level of discomfort than guilt.

Nevertheless, the non-chronic version of shame can be useful when experienced in a tiny dose.

Shame motivates you to take a good look at yourself and make radical changes to your life, rather than mindlessly heading in the wrong direction.

However, when shame becomes chronic, it turns into a self-destructive force.

Chronic shame prevents you from showing others your authentic self.

It robs you of the ability to show yourself as you are, in all your uniqueness.

How you cope with this debilitating emotional

undercurrent depends on whether your solar plexus chakra is underactive or overactive.

UNDERACTIVE SOLAR PLEXUS CHAKRA

- Weak will
- Easy to manipulate
- Poor self-esteem
- Victim mindset
- Inability to stand your ground
- Hiding from the world

If your solar plexus chakra is underactive, chronic shame shows up as a tendency to hide from the world.

This includes avoiding challenges and responsibilities.

A person with an underactive solar plexus chakra has low energy and a weak will.

They cannot stand their ground and avoid conflict at all cost.

They often exhibit a victim mindset in relation to those elements of their life they dislike.

As they cannot solve their own problems, they

often expect other people to step in and sort out these problems for them.

Alternatively, they blame fate, bad luck, or external circumstances for their discomfort.

They see themselves as powerless to institute any kind of change.

People with an underactive solar plexus chakra fear being visible and are terrified of becoming the center of ridicule.

They therefore do everything possible to avoid humiliation, often at the cost of their self-respect.

While keeping themselves powerless, they build up resentment they can only express privately.

As such, the issues that bother them tend to linger as they cannot find a way to resolve them.

UNDERACTIVE SOLAR PLEXUS CHAKRA HEALING

To heal an underactive solar plexus chakra, you need to start bringing extra energy into this area.

This means, as a first step, getting your body used to not hiding when you are out and about.

Instead, you need to allow yourself to be fully present and visible.

At a deeper level, you can heal your underactive solar plexus chakra by reminding yourself of your past successes.

This continuous act of positive remembering will boost your self-confidence.

In turn, this will nourish your solar plexus chakra in a healthy way.

UNDERACTIVE SOLAR PLEXUS CHAKRA EXERCISES

Super(wo)man pose

One of the easiest ways to bring more energy into your solar plexus chakra is to spend at least a couple of minutes at the start of your day in the so-called 'super(wo)man pose'.

This pose consists of standing with your legs spread a hip-width apart and your hands on your hips, staring straight ahead.

In adopting this pose, you are making your body bigger, which is what those who have just won a competition often do instinctively.

This physical posture gives your body the message 'you are a winner'.

This mindset strengthens your solar plexus chakra.

The effects of the super(wo)man pose were demonstrated by psychology researcher Amy Cuddy.

Her experimental studies show that our body language impacts how we think and feel about ourselves.

In one of her studies, participants sat either in the super(wo)man pose or in a low-power pose (leaning inward, legs crossed) for two minutes.

The results showed that those participants who sat in the super(wo)man pose felt more powerful and performed better in mock interviews than the participants in the low-power pose group.

In another study, Amy Cuddy also demonstrated that power posing changed the body chemistry of participants, particularly in terms of hormones.

Participants who did power posing had an increase in testosterone and a decrease in cortisol.

Both of these effects are linked with self-confidence.

Try doing the super(wo)man pose for a couple of minutes at the beginning of each day for a week and watch your confidence levels increase.

Also, the more frequently you do this pose, the better.

Use this pose as many times as you like.

This pose will do wonders for healing your underactive solar plexus chakra.

Develop a success archive

Having an underactive solar plexus chakra brings up feelings of being a fraud, not being enough as you are, or any number of other negative ways of seeing yourself.

To replace this negative self-image with a healthy sense of self, it is helpful to put together a 'success archive' for yourself.

Your success archive is a list of past successes or things that make you feel good about yourself.

If you have received any awards or other outward achievements, put them on your list.

Don't forget to list personal qualities you may have, such as kindness, compassion, and wisdom.

We are all unique and amazing in our own way, if we only spend a bit of time to think about it.

Put this list somewhere you can easily access it.

Keep coming back to your success archive as many times as you need.

Don't forget to update it as you identify more things you feel proud of.

OVERACTIVE SOLAR PLEXUS CHAKRA

- Overly aggressive
- Domineering and controlling
- Need to be right and have the last word
- Prone to anger and violence
- Stubborn

When your solar plexus chakra is overactive, it means too much energy is stored in this chakra.

Your solar plexus chakra is connected to your will and your ego.

As such, too much energy in this center tends to make you overly aggressive in the way you show up in the world and pursue your goals.

A person with an overactive solar plexus chakra tends to be domineering.

They feel the need to be right and prove themselves at every opportunity.

They are also prone to anger and impose their will on others without listening to their opinion.

As a result, they often find themselves in situations of conflict, which they often 'win' at the expense of their connection to others.

OVERACTIVE SOLAR PLEXUS CHAKRA HEALING

The easiest way to bring your overactive solar plexus chakra back to balance is to do high-energy physical exercises.

This will clear out your excess solar plexus chakra energy and allow you to do the deeper inner work required to heal this particular imbalance.

To heal at a deeper level, it is important to understand that what might look like confidence is in fact an attempt to cover up your insecurities.

The antidote is to learn how to give yourself the acknowledgement you need.

Once you learn this skill, you will no longer push as hard to get acknowledgement from others.

As a result, your relationships with others will improve.

Learning how to truly see yourself will create a secure sense of confidence.

This will provide a solid foundation for your sense of self.

OVERACTIVE SOLAR PLEXUS CHAKRA EXERCISES

Channel excess energy into physical activity

It is a common misconception that having lots of energy is always a good thing.

In fact, having too much energy with no clear focus often leads to a whole range of self-sabotaging behaviors.

When this excess energy is in your solar plexus chakra, it can become particularly destructive.

Solar plexus chakra energy needs to find release in the outside world.

When you do not have a way to release it, this energy does not disappear.

Instead, as this is solar plexus chakra energy, it encourages you to push your way into the limelight, usually in a way that damages your relationships.

Pushing your way into the limelight might show up as picking a fight with your best friend or going on an angry rant on social media.

This energy is aggressive and you often end up regretting the actions you take when this energy is upon you.

Therefore, if you have an overactive solar

plexus chakra, you need to regularly release this excess energy through physical activity.

I particularly recommend doing as many high-energy cardio exercises it takes to tire yourself out.

Feeling physically tired will allow you to transition into a mellower way of being.

Once the excess energy is out of your system for the day, you will no longer seek to push yourself out into the world.

Instead, you will surrender more easily to the flow of life.

This includes connecting through your heart instead of your ego.

Connect with your energetic essence

This exercise will help you heal your overactive solar plexus chakra at a deeper level.

It will allow you to identify and acknowledge your positive qualities in a way that provides nuance and detail.

This will enable you to truly see yourself and not require as much attention from others.

To begin with, it is important to understand that as you are born, you bring a set of qualities into the world.

Imagine that these qualities are clothes hanging on a rack.

Spend some time considering, what are the qualities that are hanging on your particular rack of clothes?

Here are some of mine: I am adventurous, curious, and great at making people feel good about themselves.

I am also optimistic and at times extremely serious.

I bring these qualities into the world every time I choose to truly show up.

What about your set of qualities? How many can you name?

Once you have identified a handful of your qualities, watch them hang on your rack of clothes.

Spend some time looking at them as a group, admiring all the light they bring into the world.

Now take one of these qualities and put it on, as if it were a piece of clothing.

What do you experience when you only wear this particular quality?

Connect with how this quality feels in your body when you are experiencing it on its own.

Now try embodying each of your qualities one by one.

Take each quality off the rack and put it on.

Allow yourself time to appreciate how your body feels when you wear that particular quality.

As a final step, put on all your qualities at the same time and allow them to melt into your body.

How does that feel?

What you are experiencing, now you are wearing all of your unique qualities in a conscious way, is your energetic essence.

This energetic essence is unique to you.

No other person brings the same combination of qualities as you.

The more connected you become to your energetic essence, the less you will need outside validation.

Practice going through each of your qualities one at a time, and then all together, as often as you like.

Over time, you will also learn to identify the unique qualities other people embody.

This recognition will seep into your interactions and imbue them with warmth and appreciation for those you are interacting with.

This will draw people magnetically to you, as they will feel good in your presence.

HEART CHAKRA

ABOUT YOUR HEART CHAKRA

Your heart chakra is located near your heart, in the center of your chest.

Its energy also connects to your thymus gland as well as your arms and hands.

This is the energy within you that motivates you to step beyond your individual ego and relate to other people.

When this chakra is healthy, your relationships with others are harmonious and nurturing.

This chakra allows you to put yourself in another person's shoes and get a glimpse of how they experience the world.

It enables you to feel compassion towards others and forgive their shortcomings.

This openness and generosity towards others is based on a nurturing relationship towards yourself.

A healthy heart chakra guides you towards people who are right for you, who appreciate your generosity and can reciprocate in their own way.

This chakra teaches you that healthy relationships are an exchange rather than a one-way street, a skilled dance between giving and receiving.

HEART CHAKRA PROBLEMS

Problems with your heart chakra stem from difficulties relating to yourself.

This also leads to problems in relating to others.

To gain insight into the specific ways your heart chakra problems show up, it is helpful to take a closer look at your early family environment.

Our parents and other early caregivers are the first to give us a sense of how others are likely to relate to us.

In addition, by observing our parents interact with other people, we form an early model of the way relationships are supposed to work.

This serves as a foundation for the way we relate to others later in life.

We may either copy what we saw, or attempt to define ourselves against it.

Either way, if your heart chakra is regularly out of balance, your early experiences of relating were in some way problematic.

The good news is that as you grow older, you have the opportunity to revisit the distorted view of relationships you may have picked up during your childhood.

This allows you to gain a deeper understanding of your relationships and improve the way you relate to yourself and others.

Heart chakra problems can show up in different ways, depending on whether your heart chakra is underactive or overactive.

UNDERACTIVE HEART CHAKRA

- Critical and judgmental
- Lonely, isolated, and withdrawn
- Depressed
- Fearing intimacy

If you have an underactive heart chakra, your problematic relationship with yourself shows up as intolerance of others, which is in fact underpinned by intolerance towards yourself.

An underactive heart chakra leads to social isolation.

People with an underactive heart chakra tend to avoid the company of others.

They fear intimacy and relationships.

As a result of their isolation, they may suffer from depression and feel lonely.

In extreme cases, it may seem like they are cut off from humanity as a whole.

They may also feel depleted by interactions with others, as they do not know how to connect in a heart-centered way.

UNDERACTIVE HEART CHAKRA HEALING

If you have an underactive heart chakra, there is not enough energy passing through this center on a regular basis.

As such, the first priority is to physically start bringing more energy into this chakra.

At a deeper level, the way to heal an underactive heart chakra is to nurture your 'psychic multiplicity'.

This is a fancy way to say you need to establish a relationship with aspects of yourself that you have so far suppressed.

As you then encounter these same aspects in other people, you will be more accepting of them.

This will improve the quality of your social interactions and motivate you to seek out more frequent and deeper connections with others.

UNDERACTIVE HEART CHAKRA EXERCISES

Thymus thump

One of the easiest ways to stimulate the energy flow in your heart chakra is to regularly do a 'thymus thump'.

Simply thump the middle of your chest with your fist a few times, the way gorillas beat their chest.

Take a few deep breaths after you do the this exercise, to further increase the flow of energy.

The thymus thump is amazing at activating the energy of your heart chakra in a short amount of time.

Doing this exercise will also allow you to

spread loving heart chakra energy throughout the rest of your body.

Reconnect with your rejected selves

This exercise is based on the premise that you are made up of a multiplicity of 'selves', rather than just one unitary 'I'.

You could think of these different selves as members of your 'inner village', each with their own personality and worldview.

Rejected selves are aspects of yourself you dislike, and that you have therefore suppressed in yourself over the years.

Unless you have done lots of therapy or other forms of personal development in the past, you are probably not conscious of your rejected selves.

However, the more you suppress them, the more they are likely to show up in your external reality as people you dislike.

Identifying and forming a conscious relation-ship with your rejected selves is one of the most effective ways to heal an underactive heart chakra.

Make a list of people you dislike.

Identify the specific reasons you dislike them.

Those character features you dislike are also in you.

These are your 'rejected selves'.

Because you have rejected these features in yourself, you cannot tolerate seeing them in another person.

As a result, you find it difficult to like these people.

Working with your rejected selves will soften your dislike for these people.

This does not mean you will like them, but they will no longer trigger you as badly as before.

As a result, you will find it easier to open your heart to the world outside yourself.

Even more importantly, this process will improve the relationship you have with yourself.

OVERACTIVE HEART CHAKRA

- Poor boundaries
- Overly sacrificing
- Unaware of own needs

If your heart chakra is overactive, the way your problematic relationship with yourself shows up is that you do everything in your power to preserve your relationships with significant others.

You do this even when these relationships are abusive rather than nurturing.

People with an overactive heart chakra tend to prioritize the needs of others above their own.

They are often incredibly loving and thoughtful towards others, but do not extend this love and thoughtfulness to themselves.

They also lack boundaries between themselves and others.

As such, they tend to take on other people's problems as their own.

They do not know how to separate their own needs from those of others.

OVERACTIVE HEART CHAKRA HEALING

The first thing to understand about healing an overactive heart chakra is that this type of imbalance usually takes a long time to heal.

One reason for this is that on the surface, some of the behaviors associated with having an overactive heart chakra look like generosity and an abundance of love.

As such, these behaviors are usually encouraged by those around you, who are often the beneficiaries of such behaviors.

It takes time to recognize the problems that accompany your behaviors, and to gradually change your mindset about the way you relate to others.

Please be patient with yourself as you start this process.

If you decide to go for it, the first step in healing an overactive heart chakra is to learn how to identify your own needs.

This is no small task, because people with an overactive heart chakra are often oblivious to their needs.

They are far more focused on fulfilling the needs of those around them.

The second step in healing your overactive heart chakra is to start setting boundaries when you interact with other people in your life.

This may include instances where people ask you for help.

In such situations, you need to learn to pause and consider your own needs before jumping to the rescue.

Do you have enough energy or resources to help them?

If you find that, upon such an examination, you cannot help them without suppressing your own needs, you have to learn to say 'no'.

It is important to stay firm on your position no matter how much they plead.

If you are not used to this level of assertiveness, this is likely to be excruciating the first few times you do it, especially with people you have helped in the past.

You will probably feel like a 'bad person' throughout such interactions.

However, it is important you understand that your beliefs of what constitutes a 'good person' are distorted in a way that benefits other people while leaving you depleted.

Part of healing your heart chakra is learning to undo this distortion.

You will have to learn to set healthy boundaries that allow you to be kind and nurturing towards yourself.

OVERACTIVE HEART CHAKRA EXERCISES

Identify your own needs

What do you need to be happy?

What would make you feel more comfortable and happier in this moment?

These questions may seem basic, but please do take the time to answer them for yourself.

Aim to keep these questions at the forefront of your mind as you go about your day.

The more aware you become of your needs, the more nurturing your relationship to yourself will be.

Set healthy boundaries

As you learn to identify your needs, it becomes possible to set healthy boundaries for yourself.

Be gentle on yourself as you learn this important life skill.

You are likely to get it wrong some of the time.

You might set boundaries that are too rigid, or too easily overruled by other people's arguments and emotional outbursts.

Do not beat yourself up as you go through this process.

You are having to learn a whole new way of relating to others and being social.

This takes time, patience, and lots of self-compassion.

Setting boundaries is not easily learned through books, although books can be great at pointing out some basic principles.

As you start practicing this skill, it would help to find some good role models.

Observe the way they set boundaries in their interactions with others.

You do not have to set boundaries the way they do.

This is not about copying, it is about getting an embodied sense of what works and what does not work in different scenarios.

If you do not have such people in your life already, set out to find them.

Once you identify someone who is good with setting boundaries, see if you can arrange an informal mentoring relationship.

Tell them you are trying to learn how to set boundaries and would appreciate their advice.

They may agree to quietly watch you as you interact with others, and give you feedback on the way you manage your boundaries.

Be creative with how you go about this process, and you will learn a crucial and life-changing skill.

THROAT CHAKRA

ABOUT YOUR THROAT CHAKRA

Your throat chakra is located in the area of your throat.

Its energy connects with your voice, your thyroid, and your ears.

The healthier your throat chakra, the clearer you tend to communicate.

As your throat chakra connects with your ears, a healthy throat chakra also makes you a good listener.

The energy of your throat chakra allows you to express your truth, to yourself and others.

It may sound odd to say the throat chakra allows you to express your truth to yourself.

However, nowadays we are surrounded by so many different energies, being able to articulate your truth to yourself is a real skill.

A healthy throat chakra gives you a sense of when it is time to talk and when it is time to listen.

This includes listening to your inner voice, instead of prioritizing the opinion of others over your own.

THROAT CHAKRA PROBLEMS

Throat chakra problems stem, at a fundamental level, from being disconnected from your own truth.

When healthy, your throat chakra acts like a 'translation device' that fulfills two important functions.

The first function is that it gathers all the 'voices' of your first four chakras: your root, sacral, solar plexus, and heart chakra.

These are the chakras most intimately connected with your body and therefore with your embodied experience.

The second function is that your throat chakra creates a synthesis of all these voices and expresses it into the wider world.

However, when there are problems with the throat chakra, at least one of these functions is compromised.

As a result, what and how you communicate is not a true representation of your inner experience.

This has a number of negative consequences for your ability to express yourself and have your voice heard.

One negative consequence is that other people often sense this disconnection intuitively.

As such, they do not engage with what you say.

Your message therefore does not 'land' successfully and is not taken up and amplified by others.

In addition, people who would resonate with your authentic message do not have a chance to hear it and gravitate towards you.

By staying disconnected from your truth, you are missing the opportunity to attract like-minded people who could support and amplify your message.

The way you cope with being disconnected from your truth depends on whether your throat chakra is underactive or overactive.

UNDERACTIVE THROAT CHAKRA

- Fear of speaking in public
- Small weak voice
- Difficulty expressing your feelings
- Low energy levels

If you have an underactive throat chakra, being disconnected from your own truth shows up through an inability to express yourself, particularly in front of other people.

An underactive throat chakra is connected with a fear of speaking in public or speaking in a small weak voice.

This imbalance also leads to low energy levels, due to your throat chakra's connection to your thyroid.

Your thyroid regulates energy levels in your body, and is negatively impacted when you suppress your voice.

People who have an underactive throat chakra also find it difficult to express their feelings.

The reason for these difficulties is not, as with the other underactive chakras, that there is not enough energy passing through this center.

Your throat chakra is the smallest of the chakras, and therefore easily fills up with energy.

However, because of the smaller size of this chakra, it tends to 'clog up' if the energy in this chakra is not regularly released and expressed.

As such, the reason your throat chakra is underactive is not because of too little energy in this center.

Instead, not being able to release this energy means you do not have enough space for new energy to pass through.

UNDERACTIVE THROAT CHAKRA HEALING

The way to heal an underactive throat chakra is to release the pent-up energy that is holding everything else back from being expressed.

This is similar to a pipe that has too much debris in it.

Eventually, the pipe will get so clogged up that little else can pass through.

The way to sort out this problem is to keep the pipe as clear as possible.

This will enable what needs to pass through to do so without getting stuck.

UNDERACTIVE THROAT CHAKRA EXERCISES

Use your voice

The first step in healing an underactive throat chakra is to learn how to release the pent-up energy that has accumulated in that area of your body.

The easiest and quickest way to do that is to use your voice and make sounds.

Humming, toning, chanting, and singing are all great ways to do this.

If you don't already have a favorite among these, experiment with different ways of using your voice and see which one works best for you.

The key is to use your voice to make sounds every day, for as long as feels good.

The more you do it, the more stuck energy you clear out of your throat chakra.

This will give you more space to express yourself in the outside world.

A side benefit of doing this regularly is that using your voice supports your thyroid.

As a result, your energy levels are likely to increase.

Give humming, toning, chanting, or singing a try.

Do at least one of these activities every day for at least a week.

You'll be amazed at the results!

Release unfinished communications

At a deeper level, to heal an underactive throat chakra, you need to release so-called 'unfinished communications'.

These are things you wish you could say to somebody but don't.

There are many reasons for unfinished communications.

Sometimes you may not have the courage to tell someone how you truly feel.

Perhaps they intimidate you, or they trigger your fear of humiliation or abandonment.

You may also worry that speaking your truth will hurt the other person.

It could even be that there is no opportunity to speak to the other person, maybe because they are deceased or there is no way of reaching them.

Unfinished communications, regardless of the reason they are unfinished, present a big problem for your throat chakra.

Having a lot to say to a person and being

unable to say it is like reaching the limit of your hard drive space.

Until you get some of the existing data off, you do not have space for more data.

The particular message you cannot express gets stuck in a loop and you keep thinking about it.

To resolve this problem, you need to release these unfinished communications.

Depending on who the other person is and the particular circumstances between you, there are different ways you could go about this.

The simplest and most straightforward way is to work up the courage to say what you need to say to the person, instead of suppressing it.

However, if this is not possible, you can still find creative ways to express yourself.

This may include writing a letter you burn instead of sending, or writing what you need to say in your journal.

OVERACTIVE THROAT CHAKRA

- Talking too much
- Gossiping
- Inability to listen

- Dominating conversations
- Interrupting people

If your throat chakra is overactive, you tend to talk too much, often without saying anything of value to your listeners.

The reason for this is that you are disconnected from your own truth, and as such what you say lacks authenticity.

This can show up as 'talking for the sake of talking', which is to fill any pauses in the conversation with talk that does not actually communicate anything of value.

In some cases, you may talk to deflect attention away from an uncomfortable truth.

Alternatively, the 'talking for the sake of talking' may show up as gossip, which sets up a common bond with others while deflecting attention away from your own vulnerability.

You may also dominate conversations and push your communications on others.

This includes ignoring what other people say and frequently interrupting them.

As a result, you take up a lot of space in conversations, instead of allowing a gentle back-and-forth between yourself and others.

OVERACTIVE THROAT CHAKRA HEALING

One of the main difficulties with an overactive throat chakra is that the energy in this chakra is released too early.

As the main channel for self-expression in the body, the throat chakra 'gathers' the energies of your first four chakras before synthesizing them into a coherent message.

However, in the case of an overactive throat chakra, the tendency is to experience the first part of this process as uncomfortable.

To avoid the discomfort, you speak before these different energies have had the chance to come into a clear, articulate synthesis.

As such, the way to heal an overactive throat chakra is to learn how to tolerate this discomfort.

Specifically, you need to be patient while the different energies gather in your throat chakra.

Allow time for them to settle into a clear message before you speak.

At a deeper level, you need to find ways to clarify your thoughts and feelings before you speak.

This may involve journaling or other silent modes of self-expression.

By the time you are ready to share your experiences with others, you will be able to articulate your thoughts and feelings in a way that reflects your personal truth.

OVERACTIVE THROAT CHAKRA EXERCISES

Learn to contain energy

The first step in healing an overactive throat chakra is to become aware that while energy from your first four chakras gathers in your throat, you are likely to experience a sense of discomfort.

The next step is to learn to tolerate this temporary discomfort.

Sit with the energy in your throat chakra for a while, allowing your thoughts to settle before starting to speak.

Over time, you will become better at containing the energy before releasing it and the discomfort will subside.

In addition, others will enjoy your company more as you become a better listener.

You will learn when it is the right moment to share something, and when you should keep quiet and listen to others.

Eventually, you will experience how satisfying

it is when your message finds a 'place to land' with the other person and is received with gratitude.

Develop a regular journaling practice

Get into the habit of journaling regularly, at least once a day.

Journaling will allow you to release the energy in your throat chakra in a way that does not negatively impact your interactions with others.

You will also gain perspective on your experiences and express yourself using fewer words.

In addition, what you share will be relevant and interesting to your audience.

As your communication style improves, others will invite you to share your insights and receive what you have to say with interest and enthusiasm.

BROW CHAKRA

ABOUT YOUR BROW CHAKRA

Your brow chakra, also called your 'third eye', is located between your eyebrows.

This energy connects with your eyes and your brain.

Someone with a healthy brow chakra has clear, uncluttered thinking, and an excellent memory.

This chakra, when healthy, also allows you to remember dreams and gain insight into repetitive patterns across the whole of your life.

With the brow chakra, we leave the realm of embodied experience of the chakras below.

Instead, we enter into the land of thoughts, visions, and possibilities.

None of these have a basis in material reality when they first arise in the brow chakra.

However, through the clarity provided by this chakra, and with the help of the lower chakras, some of them can gradually be brought into existence.

The vision offered by your brow chakra reaches further than your eyesight.

It encompasses envisioning the future and providing you with insights into your past.

Due to not being constrained by material reality, your brow chakra allows you to consider different possibilities before taking the first step.

Through your brow chakra, you 'see' not only what is in front of you but also what might be possible and the circumstances that would make it so.

Your brow chakra is the wise guide you meet at the crossroads, who can help you discern the path that is right for you.

Their only request is that you take time to reflect on the different options instead of jumping into action straight away.

BROW CHAKRA PROBLEMS

Brow chakra problems stem from an inability to see clearly.

This lack of clarity is not about seeing in the physical sense.

It refers to the inability to have a clear vision for the future.

This is often accompanied by a lack of clear insight into the past.

This inability to see clearly can show up in different ways, depending on whether the brow chakra is underactive or overactive.

UNDERACTIVE BROW CHAKRA

- Difficulty envisioning the future
- Lack of imagination
- Difficulty visualizing
- Feeling stuck

If your brow chakra is underactive, there is too little energy passing through this center.

If you have an underactive brow chakra, you may miss some of the gifts of this chakra: vision, imagination, and the ability to consider different possibilities before deciding on a course of action.

You are also likely to live with little intent, largely governed by the conditioning you have picked up from your environment.

As such, making changes in your life is hard.

You may not know where to begin and feel stuck.

UNDERACTIVE BROW CHAKRA HEALING

The first step in healing an underactive brow chakra is to bring more energy into this energy center.

To do so, you need to set the intention to exercise your brow chakra on a daily basis.

You can put your brow chakra to good use by learning how to prioritize your tasks and plan out your day.

At a deeper level, the way to heal your underactive brow chakra is to spend more time engaging with the subtle aspect of existence.

This includes reading books, learning new skills, and getting into the habit of reflecting on yourself and your life.

Over time, as you become able to hold more

energy in this center, you will start envisioning change and developing more of your true potential.

UNDERACTIVE BROW CHAKRA EXERCISES

Envision your perfect day

One way to exercise your brow chakra is to use your imagination to envision the day ahead.

You may already use this forward-thinking ability unconsciously when you have anxiety-provoking scenarios running through your mind.

However, you can start taking conscious control over your brow chakra's ability to envision possible futures.

For example, if you have a meeting scheduled, take a few moments to envision every detail of that meeting going as well as it can possibly go. What would that look like?

Also envision other aspects of your day in advance, such as the great breakfast you will eat, or the walk you might take in the afternoon.

Put as much detail into your envisioning as you can and make it positive.

Most importantly, envision your day as if it has already happened.

Delight in the achievement of this perfect day

and allow yourself to feel good in every cell of your body.

The more you do this, the more you will attract positive things into your life.

Play with possibilities

Ask yourself 'what if?' questions as you go about your day.

For example, as you start work for the day, you might ask yourself, 'what if I was in a completely different job?', or 'what if instead of this job, I was working as a magician?' (assuming you are not a magician!).

Then answer the questions, allowing your imagination free rein.

The point of this exercise is to become less attached to your material day-to-day reality and allow yourself time to play with the energy of your brow chakra.

There are no wrong answers to your 'what if' questions.

The point is to get into the habit of envisioning possibilities.

OVERACTIVE BROW CHAKRA

- Difficulty concentrating
- Nightmares
- Lack of clarity
- Mental fatigue

If your brow chakra is overactive, there is too much energy passing through this center.

This overflow of energy shows up as too many thoughts running through your mind and difficulty concentrating.

You may also suffer from a general inability to prioritize and organize what is going on in your mind and in your life overall.

Your constant mental chatter gives you little space to find peace within yourself.

As your visual cortex is overly stimulated, you may also suffer from an overactive dream world.

You are likely to have a poor quality of sleep due to anxiety dreams that do not allow you to recover fully during the night.

OVERACTIVE BROW CHAKRA HEALING

The first step in healing your overactive brow chakra is to become aware of the overflow of visual images to which you are exposing your brain every day.

The problem is compounded by the fact that nowadays, this overflow is considered 'normal'.

As the world has become more mentally focused, the demands on the brow chakra have increased.

We are surrounded by screens, emails, books, and a whole range of other things that push our brain to keep working without a break.

In addition, with the arrival of the selfie and the proliferation of images online, our visual sphere is more crowded than ever.

The good news is that once you become aware of this visual overstimulation, you can do something about it.

One of the first things you can do is to declutter your environment and anything else you regularly have in front of your eyes, such as your computer desktop.

Once you are free of the overflow of visual

stimuli, you can take active steps to put your ideas in order.

In particular, you need to get into the habit of writing down your thoughts.

This will stop them from going around your mind on a loop and allow your brain time to rest.

OVERACTIVE BROW CHAKRA EXERCISES

Declutter your environment

If your brow chakra is overactive, you need to reduce the amount of mental stimulation in your environment.

This includes items such as books (and book-shelves), folders, screens, and anything that triggers your brain into working overtime.

As you are reading this, take a few moments to look around your environment.

Do you have any bookshelves within visual range?

What about other items that are mentally stim-ulating?

If you do, you need to declutter your space of mentally stimulating material.

Perhaps you can relocate your books inside a cupboard or somewhere you cannot see them.

The same goes for other items that stimulate your visual field and your brain, such as work folders.

The more simplicity you can introduce into your living and working environment, the quicker your overstimulated brow chakra can heal.

This may be tricky in situations where you have little control over your environment.

If this applies to you, I advise you to find a corner of your 'world' you do have control over.

Make this corner as visually simple as possible.

Regularly looking at an oasis of simplicity and order will allow your brow chakra to find a restful anchor.

Write things down

At a deeper level, the way to heal an overactive brow chakra is to discipline your mind and put order among your ideas.

The easiest and quickest way to do that is to write your ideas down, and to develop a process for organizing what you have written.

This will allow you to gain perspective, instead of letting your ideas swirl around in your head, disturbing your peace.

The way you organize your ideas once you have written them down has to be uniquely tailored to the way your brain works.

There is not much guidance I can offer for what this process should look like.

However, the main point of this process is to provide you with a structure, a 'container', into which you can put your thoughts.

It also has to offer you a way to later extract the information you need from that container.

Experiment with different ways of capturing and organizing your ideas.

Over time, you will discover what works best for you.

CROWN CHAKRA

ABOUT YOUR CROWN CHAKRA

Your crown chakra is located just above the top of your head.

The energy of this chakra is the most difficult to describe in clear, logical language.

Logic is not what this chakra is about.

Instead, if I was to sum up this energy in one word, it would be 'trust'.

By 'trust' I don't mean the interpersonal kind, such as trusting another person's honesty.

Crown chakra trust is of a transpersonal kind.

It is about trusting life itself and the wider forces that govern all of existence.

When you have a healthy crown chakra, you trust that life is inherently meaningful.

As such, you surrender to things as they are and the situations you are finding yourself in.

You trust that the reason you are experiencing these situations will reveal itself over time.

This trusting attitude stands in sharp contrast to the way most of us live our lives, especially the way we attempt to micro-manage every aspect of our existence.

The trust associated with the crown chakra is not based on anything material, such as having financial security or being in good health.

Instead, you trust because through this chakra you are connected to all aspects of existence.

You know that in the large scheme of things, everything is going to turn out fine.

What is meant to be will be.

You can probably sense the abstract quality that comes across as I am attempting to articulate the essence of this energy into words.

That in itself is strangely fitting.

As the crown chakra is the most 'big picture' of all the chakras, this abstract quality captures the essence of this energy.

That is perhaps the best we can hope for with this most elusive of chakras.

'Trust', a word and a feeling I have already mentioned in relation to this energy, takes us to the concept of a 'belief system'.

This is a fancy term to describe everything you believe to be true about the world.

Everyone has a belief system, whether they realize it or not.

If you were to make a list of all the things you believe to be true, you may be surprised by how many beliefs you have.

A belief system includes general beliefs such as 'people are intrinsically good' and 'life is worth living'.

It also includes beliefs about yourself, such as 'I am good with money' and 'I am resourceful'.

These beliefs trickle down from your crown chakra towards your other chakras, from top to bottom, until they 'manifest' into the tangible reality of your life.

Let's take the belief 'I am good with money'.

Imagine this belief originating in your crown chakra and then moving downwards.

Visualize the energy of this belief reaching your brow chakra, which regulates a lot of your mental processes and therefore influences your thoughts.

Once there, the belief 'I am good with money' may turn into a detailed financial plan.

This belief then trickles further into your throat chakra and influences the things you say about yourself, which may encourage others to entrust you with financial responsibilities.

Down and down this energy travels, until it reaches the physical dimension of life and shows up as your current material reality.

Can you see how your beliefs, originating in your crown chakra, influence the rest of your life?

Even though this energy is difficult to describe in words, I hope you are starting to understand how it shows up in your life.

In general, a healthy crown chakra brings extraordinary wisdom.

When you are connected with this energy, you find meaning in every aspect of your existence.

Instead of resisting what happens in your life, you gratefully surrender to it and wait for the meaning to reveal itself as events unfold.

CROWN CHAKRA PROBLEMS

As the crown chakra is so closely tied to the feeling of trust, problems with your crown chakra stem from a distorted relationship with this feeling.

We are surrounded by so many different points of view and so many sources of information nowadays.

How can we distinguish what to believe and whom to trust?

This uncertainty around trust affects our inner sense of knowing and therefore our ability to make decisions that are good for us.

The way you cope with crown chakra difficulties depends on whether this chakra is underactive or overactive.

UNDERACTIVE CROWN CHAKRA

- Cynicism
- Rigid belief system
- Apathy
- Difficulty finding meaning

If your crown chakra is underactive, your problematic relationship with trust shows up as a generalized mistrust.

You therefore tend to close down this chakra to anything coming in from the outside.

The way you deal with outside information that contradicts your own beliefs is to dismiss it without giving it any consideration.

The problem is that in doing so, you close yourself off from revising your existing beliefs, many of which may be outdated.

As a child, you soaked up your family's beliefs without giving them any consideration. You had no choice.

However, as an adult, you have the opportunity to revise your beliefs.

You can decide which ones are worth keeping and which ones no longer hold true.

It is your crown chakra that is most helpful in this process, as it allows you to come into contact with new, more empowering beliefs.

However, if your crown chakra is underactive, it cannot perform this function, so you remain stuck with your outdated beliefs.

This feeling of stuckness is also linked to boredom and apathy.

As the crown chakra helps you find meaning in

your life, too little energy in this area leads to living in a disenchanted way.

You are therefore likely to suffer from low mood and a general numbness to all the wonders life has to offer.

UNDERACTIVE CROWN CHAKRA HEALING

The way to heal an underactive crown chakra is to consciously examine your beliefs.

This will enable you to identify and challenge your limiting beliefs.

These are beliefs that are likely to have come from your environment while growing up and no longer hold true in your current reality.

Instead, they are holding you back from realizing your full potential.

At a deeper level, the way to heal an underactive crown chakra is to start looking at the big picture of your life.

How do the activities in your day-to-day life fit into this bigger picture?

If your life was a story, what kind of hero would you be?

What story would you be telling?

Asking yourself these big picture questions will infuse your daily life with meaning and inspiration.

UNDERACTIVE CROWN CHAKRA EXERCISES

Revise your existing beliefs

Every time you hear yourself saying something about yourself or about the way things are, take a few moments to consider what you have just said.

Ask yourself a couple of simple questions in relation to this belief.

Is this actually true?

Is this belief empowering?

For example, take a belief that often gets passed down through the generations and that you may hold true: 'life is hard'.

You will probably find that this belief did indeed hold true for many of your ancestors, perhaps due to food shortages and many other physical constraints.

However, what if this belief did not have to hold true for you?

The problem is that if you hold this belief, it trickles down and influences the energy of your other chakras.

As such, the reality you bring into existence continuously reflects this belief back to you.

What if you could replace this disempowering belief with 'life is fun'?

You can go through this process with any of your beliefs.

See if they still hold true for you, and if they are empowering or disempowering.

Disempowering beliefs prevent you from living out your true potential.

As you keep going through this process, you will discover more limiting beliefs.

Make a list of these beliefs.

Write at least one empowering alternative next to each of your limiting beliefs.

Once you are happy with the wording of your empowering alternatives, write these again on a separate list.

Put this list in a place that is visible to you, especially as you go to bed at night and wake up in the morning.

You can also record these empowering alternatives as affirmations and listen to them as you drift off to sleep.

Over time, your limiting beliefs will dissolve,

and your physical reality will start improving as a result.

Look for meaning

How open are you to the idea that life is meaningful?

Can you see how every event in your life, every decision you have taken, has brought you to this present moment?

At every turn, your soul is guiding you towards more growth at the spiritual level.

Start paying attention to the things you see and hear over the course of your day.

Consider the possibility that these are messages from your soul.

As you pay attention to the guidance you receive in this seemingly random way, you will get more help in navigating your life.

OVERACTIVE CROWN CHAKRA

- Attempting to escape material concerns
- Highly suggestible

- Poor attention to detail
- Pulled in different directions
- Difficulty getting things done

If your crown chakra is overactive, your distorted relationship with trust leads you to get pulled into the vortex of other people's thoughts and beliefs.

You are likely to trust information you gather from the outside world too easily, without passing it through the filter of your own experience.

You may also waste your time thinking about things that are not relevant to you and be too distracted to get things done.

An overactive crown chakra may also show up as living with your 'head in the clouds', not taking an interest in the material aspects of life that require your attention.

As a result, urgent material concerns such as unpaid bills are likely to pile up and become overwhelming.

OVERACTIVE CROWN CHAKRA HEALING

Healing an overactive crown chakra is about filtering the thoughts, information, and beliefs you take in from other people.

Over time, you will discard anything that is not relevant or trustworthy.

Instead, you will put your energy into the things that can help you turn your dreams into reality.

At a deeper level, healing your overactive crown chakra is about learning how to live your life in a more grounded way.

Stop dismissing the mundane matters of life in pursuit of intellectual or spiritual matters.

Instead, start taking an active involvement in mundane matters.

Over time, this will make your day-to-day experiences meaningful and enjoyable.

OVERACTIVE CROWN CHAKRA EXERCISES

Filter incoming information

The first step in healing an overactive crown chakra is to develop a filtering process for any outside information you receive.

Ask yourself, how is this relevant to me right now?

Is this actually true? What is my own experience?

Who is this information coming from? Can I trust this source?

Is this the right time to put my energy into this?

The more you get into the habit of filtering the information you take in, the easier it will be to bring focus into your life.

Focus on mundane matters

One of the gifts you already possess with an overactive crown chakra is that you see everything as connected and meaningful.

However, the problem is that you use this gift to bypass the mundane matters of life.

To heal your overactive crown chakra, you need to learn to stay present when mundane matters present themselves.

Such matters include a blocked toilet, an unpaid bill, or other practical tasks.

Ask yourself, what mundane aspects of life are you attempting to avoid by keeping your crown chakra overactive?

The mundane aspect of existence is where your growth is.

You need to find solid ground underneath your feet.

This solid ground will act as a container for the amazing inspiration you are gathering through your crown chakra.

The more you stay present with the mundane instead of attempting to avoid it, the more you infuse the mundane with wonder and meaning.

CONCLUSION

I hope this book has provided you with clarity on how to use your chakras to identify aspects of your life that need extra attention.

I also hope you have found useful suggestions on what you can do to address these areas of your life.

Over the course of this book, you have probably come across chakras where you identified with both the underactive as well as the overactive aspect.

As mentioned in the introduction, this is often the case with some chakras.

Energy is in constant flux. As such, it is no wonder the energy in our chakras fluctuates too.

As you start engaging with these chakras that

are both under- and overactive, you will learn to recognize where you are at any given moment on that continuum.

It is your awareness that is the most important when working with your chakras.

The more you become aware of your own patterns, and of the distortions that lie beneath some of them, the more you gain conscious control of your life.

Over time, you will no longer be tossed here and there by the currents of everyday existence.

You can then start using your energy productively and fulfill your true potential. And that is worth celebrating!

The more you work with the energy of your chakras, the more your understanding of what they represent will evolve.

Be prepared for this change and stay open-minded as more insights come into your awareness.

Healing your chakras is an ongoing process, so please be patient with yourself.

Treat this as a journey of exploration and curiosity rather than as a finite goal.

I wish you all the best in this extraordinary journey of self-discovery.

I would like to ask you for a small favor.

Reviews are the best way to spread the word about this book.

If you have found this book helpful, it would mean a lot to me if you could leave a review.

Even if you only write a sentence or two, it will help. Thank you!

ABOUT THE AUTHOR

Alexa Ispas holds a PhD in psychology from the University of Edinburgh and had originally planned to become an academic.

A series of unexpected events led her to experience energy healing.

This extraordinary form of healing had a profound impact on her perception of the world and her place within it.

Becoming aware of the way her energy functions provided Alexa with a filter through which she could evaluate and transform every aspect of her life.

Over the next several years, Alexa trained and worked as an energy healer.

During this time, she used her psychology background to develop a practical and down-to-earth approach to energy work.

This approach forms the basis for the books in her *Energy Awareness Series*.

The series aims to help readers at all levels

understand how their energy works and how to interact with the subtle dimension of life.

If you'd like to stay in touch with Alexa and learn more about energy awareness, please sign up to her newsletter.

As a small 'thank you', you will receive a free book when you sign up.

You can sign up to the newsletter and receive your free book at www.alexaispas.com/newsletter

NOURISH YOUR CHAKRAS

Chakras are well-known for leading to deep personal transformation, but do you know how to take care of yours?

In *Nourish Your Chakras*, energy healer Alexa Ispas teaches you one simple thing you can do to look after each of your chakras every day.

Download for free when you sign up to Alexa's newsletter at

www.alexaispas.com/newsletter

Printed in Great Britain
by Amazon